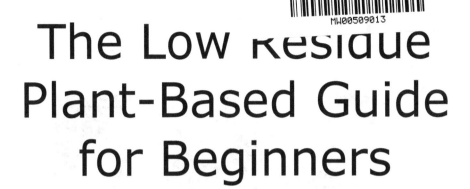

The Low Residue Plant-Based Guide for Beginners

A Comprehensive Plant-Based Diet Guide for Healthy People

Levi Tonge

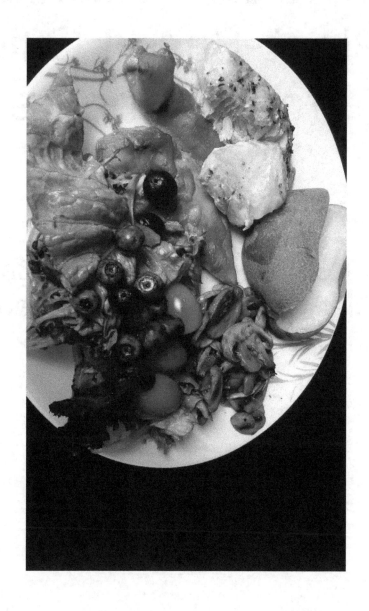

from various sources. Please consult a licensed professional before attempting any techniques outlined in this book.

By reading this document, the reader agrees that under no circumstances is the author responsible for any losses, direct or indirect, which are incurred as a result of the use of information contained within this document, including, but not limited to, — errors, omissions, or inaccuracies.

Table of Contents

Hazelnut And Chocolate Milk

Servings: 2

Cooking Time: 0 Minute

Ingredients:

- 2 tablespoons cocoa powder
- 4 dates, pitted
- 1 cup hazelnuts
- 3 cups of water

Directions:

1. Place all the ingredients in the order in a food processor or blender and then pulse for 2 to 3 minutes at high speed until smooth.

2. Pour the smoothie into two glasses and then serve.

Nutrition Info: Calories: 120 Cal; Fat: 5 g: Carbs: 19 g; Protein: 2 g; Fiber: 1 g

Bean & Spinach Casserole

Servings: 6

Cooking Time: 35 Minutes

Ingredients:

- 3 tbsp olive oil
- 1 onion, chopped
- 2 carrots, chopped
- 1 celery stalk, chopped
- 2 garlic cloves, minced
- 1 (15.5-oz) can Navy beans
- 1 (15.5-oz) can Great Northern beans
- 1 cup baby spinach
- 3 tomatoes, chopped
- 1 cup vegetable broth
- 1 tbsp fresh parsley, chopped
- 1 tsp dried thyme
- Salt and black pepper to taste
- ½ cup breadcrumbs

Directions:

1. Preheat oven to 380 F.

2.   Heat the oil in a skillet over medium heat. Place in onion, carrots, celery, and garlic. Sauté for 5 minutes. Remove into a greased casserole. Add in beans, spinach, tomatoes, broth, parsley, thyme, salt, and pepper and stir to combine. Cover with foil and bake in the oven for 15 minutes.

3.   Next, take out the casserole from the oven, remove the foil and spread the breadcrumbs all over. Bake for another 10 minutes until the top is crispy and golden. Serve warm.

Mediterranean-style Zucchini Pancakes

Servings: 4

Cooking Time: 20 Minutes

Ingredients:

- 1 cup all-purpose flour
- 1/2 teaspoon baking powder
- 1/2 teaspoon dried oregano
- 1/2 teaspoon dried basil
- 1/2 teaspoon dried rosemary
- Sea salt and ground black pepper, to taste
- 1 ½ cups zucchini, grated
- 1 chia egg
- 1/2 cup rice milk
- 1 teaspoon garlic, minced
- 2 tablespoons scallions, sliced
- 4 tablespoons olive oil

Directions:

1. Thoroughly combine the flour, baking powder and spices. In a separate bowl, combine the zucchini, chia egg, milk, garlic and scallions.

2.   Add the zucchini mixture to the dry flour mixture; stir to combine well.

3.   Then, heat the olive oil in a frying pan over a moderate flame. Cook your pancakes for 2 to minutes per side until golden brown.

4.   Bon appétit!

Nutrition Info: Per Serving: Calories: 260; Fat: 14.1g; Carbs: 27.1g; Protein: 4.6g

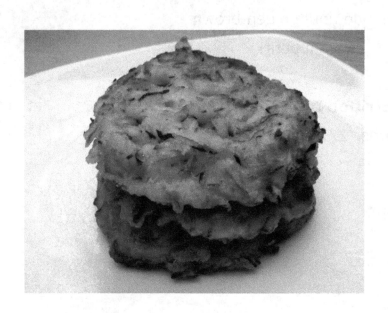

Chocolate Mint Smoothie

Servings: 1

Cooking Time: 5 Minutes

Ingredients:

- 2 tbsp. sweetener of your choice
- 2 drops mint extract
- 1 tbsp. cocoa powder
- ½ avocado, medium
- ¼ c. coconut milk
- 1 c. almond milk, unsweetened

Directions:

1. In a high-speed blender, add all the ingredients and blend until smooth.
2. Add two to four ice cubes and blend.
3. Serve immediately and enjoy!

Nutrition Info: Calories: 401 Carbohydrates: 6.3 g Proteins: 5 g Fats: 40.3 g

Traditional Hanukkah Latkes

Servings: 6

Cooking Time: 30 Minutes

Ingredients:

- 1 ½ pounds potatoes, peeled, grated and drained
- 3 tablespoons green onions, sliced
- 1/3 cup all-purpose flour
- 1/2 teaspoon baking powder
- 1/2 teaspoon sea salt, preferably kala namak
- 1/4 teaspoon ground black pepper
- 1/2 olive oil
- 5 tablespoons applesauce
- 1 tablespoon fresh dill, roughly chopped

Directions:

1.   Thoroughly combine the grated potato, green onion, flour, baking powder, salt and black pepper.

2.   Preheat the olive oil in a frying pan over a moderate heat.

3.   Spoon 1/4 cup of potato mixture into the pan and cook your latkes until golden brown on both sides. Repeat with the remaining batter.

4.   Serve with applesauce and fresh dill. Bon appétit!

Nutrition Info: Per Serving: Calories: 283; Fat: 18.4g; Carbs: 27.3g; Protein: 3.2g

Fragrant Spiced Coffee

Servings: 8

Cooking Time: 3 Hours

Ingredients:

- 4 cinnamon sticks, each about 3 inches long
- 1 1/2 teaspoons of whole cloves
- 1/3 cup of honey
- 2-ounce of chocolate syrup
- 1/2 teaspoon of anise extract
- 8 cups of brewed coffee

Directions:

1.   Pour the coffee in a 4-quarts slow cooker and pour in the remaining ingredients except for cinnamon and stir properly.

2.   Wrap the whole cloves in cheesecloth and tie its corners with strings.

3.   Immerse this cheesecloth bag in the liquid present in the slow cooker and cover it with the lid.

4.   Then plug in the slow cooker and let it cook on the low heat setting for 3 hours or until heated thoroughly.

5.   When done, discard the cheesecloth bag and serve.

Nutrition Info: Calories:150 Cal, Carbohydrates:35g, Protein:3g, Fats:0g, Fiber:0g.

Ambrosia Salad with Pecans

Servings: 4

Cooking Time: 15 Minutes

Ingredients:

- 1 cup pure coconut cream
- ½ tsp vanilla extract
- 2 medium bananas, peeled and cut into chunks
- 1 ½ cups unsweetened coconut flakes
- 4 tbsp toasted pecans, chopped
- 1 cup pineapple tidbits, drained
- 1 (11 oz) can mandarin oranges, drained
- ¾ cup maraschino cherries, stems removed

Directions:

1.   In medium bowl, mix the coconut cream and vanilla extract until well combined.

2.   In a larger bowl, combine the bananas, coconut flakes, pecans, pineapple, oranges, and cherries until evenly distributed.

3.   Pour on the coconut cream mixture and fold well into the salad.

4. Chill in the refrigerator for 1 hour and serve afterwards.

Nutrition Info: al info per serving: Calories 648; Fats 36g; Carbs 85.7g; Protein 6.6g

Homemade Apple Butter

Servings: 16

Cooking Time: 35 Minutes

Ingredients:

*   5 pounds apples, peeled, cored and diced
*   1 cup water
*   2/3 cup granulated brown sugar
*   1 tablespoon ground cinnamon
*   1 teaspoon ground cloves
*   1 tablespoon vanilla essence
*   A pinch of freshly grated nutmeg
*   A pinch of salt

Directions:

1.   Add the apples and water to a heavy-bottomed pot and cook for about 20 minutes.

2.   Then, mash the cooked apples with a potato masher; stir the sugar, cinnamon, cloves, vanilla, nutmeg and salt into the mashed apples; stir to combine well.

3.   Continue to simmer until the butter has thickened to your desired consistency.

4.   Bon appétit!

Nutrition Info: Per Serving: Calories: 106; Fat: 0.3g; Carbs: 27.3g; Protein: 0.4g

White Chocolate Pudding

Servings: 4

Cooking Time: 4 Hours 20 Minutes

Ingredients:

- 3 tbsp flax seed + 9 tbsp water
- 3 tbsp cornstarch
- ¼ tbsp salt
- 1 cup cashew cream
- 2 ½ cups almond milk
- ½ pure date sugar
- 1 tbsp vanilla caviar
- 6 oz unsweetened white chocolate chips
- Whipped coconut cream for topping
- Sliced bananas and raspberries for topping

Directions:

1.   In a small bowl, mix the flax seed powder with water and allow thickening for 5 minutes to make the flax egg.

2.   In a large bowl, whisk the cornstarch and salt, and then slowly mix in the in the cashew cream until smooth. Whisk in the flax egg until well combined.

3.   Pour the almond milk into a pot and whisk in the date sugar. Cook over medium heat while frequently stirring until the sugar dissolves. Reduce the heat to low and simmer until steamy and bubbly around the edges.

4.   Pour half of the almond milk mixture into the flax egg mix, whisk well and pour this mixture into the remaining milk content in the pot. Whisk continuously until well combined.

5.   Bring the new mixture to a boil over medium heat while still frequently stirring and scraping all the corners of the pot, 2 minutes.

6.   Turn the heat off, stir in the vanilla caviar, then the white chocolate chips until melted. Spoon the mixture into a bowl, allow cooling for 2 minutes, cover with plastic wraps making sure to press the plastic onto the surface of the pudding, and refrigerate for 4 hours.

7.   Remove the pudding from the fridge, take off the plastic wrap and whip for about a minute.

8.   Spoon the dessert into serving cups, swirl some coconut whipping cream on top, and top with the bananas and raspberries. Enjoy immediately.

Nutrition Info: al infoper serving: Calories 654; Fats 47.9g; Carbs 52.1g; Protein 7.3g

Oat Porridge with Almonds

Servings: 2

Cooking Time: 20 Minutes

Ingredients:

- 1 cup water
- 2 cups almond milk, divided
- 1 cup rolled oats
- 2 tablespoons coconut sugar
- 1/2 vanilla essence
- 1/4 teaspoon cardamom
- 1/2 cup almonds, chopped
- 1 banana, sliced

Directions:

1. In a deep saucepan, bring the water and milk to a rapid boil. Add in the oats, cover the saucepan and turn the heat to medium.

2. Add in the coconut sugar, vanilla and cardamom. Continue to cook for about 1minutes, stirring periodically.

3.   Spoon the mixture into serving bowls; top with almonds and banana. Bon appétit!

Nutrition Info: Per Serving: Calories: 533; Fat: 13.7g; Carbs: 85g; Protein: 21.6g

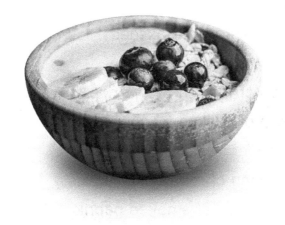

Southwest Spinach Salad

Servings: 2

Cooking Time: 10 Minutes

Ingredients:

- ½ a tablespoon of flaxseeds
- ½ a cup of corn
- ½ a cup of cooked brown rice
- ½ a cup of cooked black beans
- 8 ounces of fresh spinach
- ¼ teaspoon of red pepper flakes
- ½ a teaspoon of smoked paprika
- ½ a teaspoon of BBQ sauce
- ½ a teaspoon of balsamic vinegar

Directions:

1. Combine the BBQ sauce, red pepper flakes, paprika and vinegar in a large bowl and whisk to combine.

2. Add the corn, rice, black beans and spinach and toss to coat.

3. Divide onto plates, top with flaxseed and serve.

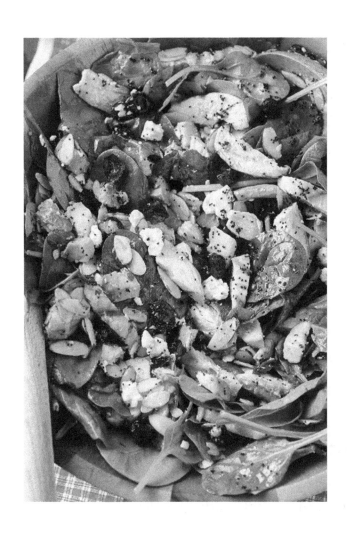

Oat & Chickpea Burgers with Avocado Dip

Servings: 4

Cooking Time: 20 Minutes

Ingredients:

- 1 large avocado, pitted and peeled
- 1 tomato, chopped
- 1 small red onion, chopped
- 3 (15 oz) cans chickpeas, drained
- 2 tbsp almond flour
- 2 tbsp quick-cooking oats
- ¼ cup chopped fresh parsley
- 1 tbsp hot sauce
- 1 garlic clove, minced
- ¼ tsp garlic salt
- 1/8 tsp black pepper
- 4 whole-grain hamburger buns, split

Directions:

1.   In a medium bowl, mash avocados and mix in the tomato and onion. Set aside the dip.

2.   In another bowl, mash the chickpeas and mix in the almond flour, oats, parsley, hot sauce, garlic, garlic salt, and black pepper. Mold 4 patties out of the mixture and set aside.

3.   Heat a grill pan to medium heat and lightly grease with cooking spray. Cook the bean patties on both sides until light brown and cooked through, 10 minutes. Place each patty between each burger bun and top with the avocado dip.

Oriental Bulgur & White Beans

Servings: 4

Cooking Time: 55 Minutes

Ingredients:

- 2 tbsp olive oil
- 3 green onions, chopped
- 1 cup bulgur
- 1 cups water
- 1 tbsp soy sauce
- Salt to taste
- 1 ½ cups cooked white beans
- 1 tbsp nutritional yeast
- 1 tbsp dried parsley

Directions:

1.   Heat the oil in a pot over medium heat. Place in green onions and sauté for 3 minutes. Stir in bulgur, water, soy sauce, and salt. Bring to a boil, then lower the heat and simmer for 20-22 minutes. Mix in beans and yeast. Cook for 5 minutes. Serve topped with parsley.

Veggie Noodles

Servings: 2

Cooking Time: 5 Minutes

Ingredients:

- 2 tablespoons vegetable oil
- 4 spring onions, divided
- 1 cup snap pea
- 2 tablespoons brown sugar
- 9 oz. dried rice noodles, cooked
- 5 garlic cloves, minced
- 2 carrots, cut into small sticks
- 3 tablespoons soy sauce

Directions:

1. Heat vegetable oil in a skillet over medium heat and add garlic and 3 spring onions.
2. Cook for about 3 minutes and add the carrots, peas, brown sugar and soy sauce.
3. Add rice noodles and cook for about 2 minutes.
4. Season with salt and black pepper and top with remaining spring onion to serve.

Rich Truffle Hot Chocolate

Servings: 4

Cooking Time: 2 Hours

Ingredients:

- 1/3 cup of cocoa powder, unsweetened
- 1/3 cup of coconut sugar
- 1/8 teaspoon of salt
- 1/8 teaspoon of ground cinnamon
- 1 teaspoon of vanilla extract, unsweetened
- 32 fluid ounce of coconut milk

Directions:

1.   Using a 2 quarts slow cooker, add all the ingredients and stir properly.

2.   Cover it with the lid, then plug in the slow cooker and cook it for hours on the high heat setting or until it is heated thoroughly.

3.   When done, serve right away.

Nutrition Info: Calories:67 Cal, Carbohydrates:13g, Protein:2g, Fats:2g, Fiber:2.3g.

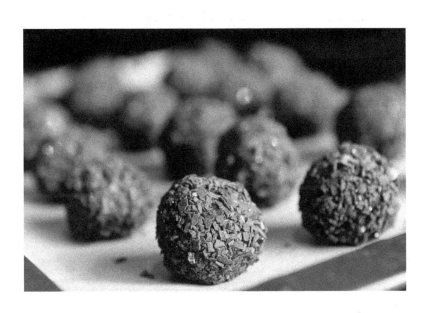

Celery Buckwheat Croquettes

Servings: 6

Cooking Time: 25 Minutes

Ingredients:

- ¾ cup cooked buckwheat groats
- ½ cup cooked brown rice
- 3 tbsp olive oil
- ¼ cup minced onion
- 1 celery stalk, chopped
- ¼ cup shredded carrots
- 1/3 cup whole-wheat flour
- ¼ cup chopped fresh parsley
- Salt and black pepper to taste

Directions:

1. Combine the groats and rice in a bowl. Set aside. Heat tbsp of oil in a skillet over medium heat. Place in onion, celery and carrot and cook for 5 minutes. Transfer to the rice bowl. Mix in flour, parsley, salt, and pepper. Place in the fridge for 20 minutes. Mould the mixture into cylinder-shaped balls.

2.   Heat the remaining oil in a skillet over medium heat. Fry the croquettes for 8 minutes, turning occasionally until golden. Serve warm.

Apple And Cranberry Chutney

Servings: 7

Cooking Time: 1 Hour

Ingredients:

- 1 ½ pounds cooking apples, peeled, cored and diced
- 1/2 cup sweet onion, chopped
- 1/2 cup apple cider vinegar
- 1 large orange, freshly squeezed
- 1 cup brown sugar
- 1 teaspoon fennel seeds
- 1 tablespoon fresh ginger, peeled and grated
- 1 teaspoon sea salt
- 1/2 cup dried cranberries

Directions:

1. In a saucepan, place the apples, sweet onion, vinegar, orange juice, brown sugar, fennel seeds, ginger and salt. Bring the mixture to a boil.

2. Immediately turn the heat to simmer; continue to simmer, stirring occasionally, for approximately 55 minutes, until most of the liquid has absorbed.

3. Set aside to cool and add in the dried cranberries. Store in your refrigerator for up to 2 weeks.

4. Bon appétit!

Nutrition Info: Per Serving: Calories: 208; Fat: 0.3g; Carbs: 53g; Protein: 0.6g

Warm Pomegranate Punch

Servings: 10

Cooking Time: 3 Hours

Ingredients:

- 3 cinnamon sticks, each about 3 inches long
- 12 whole cloves
- 1/2 cup of coconut sugar
- 1/3 cup of lemon juice
- 32 fluid ounce of pomegranate juice
- 32 fluid ounce of apple juice, unsweetened
- 16 fluid ounce of brewed tea

Directions:

1. Using a 4-quart slow cooker, pour the lemon juice, pomegranate, juice apple juice, tea, and then sugar.

2. Wrap the whole cloves and cinnamon stick in a cheese cloth, tie its corners with a string, and immerse it in the liquid present in the slow cooker.

3. Then cover it with the lid, plug in the slow cooker and let it cook at the low heat setting for hours or until it is heated thoroughly.

4.   When done, discard the cheesecloth bag and serve it hot or cold.

Nutrition Info: Calories:253 Cal, Carbohydrates:58g, Protein:7g, Fats:2g, Fiber:3g.

Spaghetti in Spicy Tomato Sauce

Servings: 4

Cooking Time: 40 Minutes

Ingredients:

- 1 pound dried spaghetti
- 1 red bell pepper, diced
- 4 garlic cloves, minced
- 1 teaspoon red pepper flakes, crushed
- 2 (14-ounce) cans diced tomatoes
- 1 (6-ounce) can tomato paste
- 2 teaspoons vegan sugar, granulated
- 2 tablespoons olive oil
- 1 medium onion, diced
- 1 cup dry red wine
- 1 teaspoon dried thyme
- ½ teaspoon fennel seed, crushed
- 1½ cups coconut milk, full-fat
- Salt and black pepper, to taste

Directions:

1. Boil water in a large pot and add pasta.

2. Cook according to the package directions and drain the pasta into a colander.

3. Dish out the pasta in a large serving bowl and add a dash of olive oil to prevent sticking.

4. Heat 2 tablespoons of olive oil over medium heat in a large pot and add garlic, onion and bell pepper.

5. Sauté for about minutes and stir in the wine, thyme, fennel and red pepper flakes.

6. Allow to simmer on high heat for about 5 minutes until the liquid is reduced by about half.

7. Add diced tomatoes and tomato paste and allow to simmer for about 20 minutes, stirring occasionally.

8. Stir in the coconut milk and sugar and simmer for about 10 more minutes.

9. Season with salt and black pepper and pour the sauce over the pasta.

10. Toss to coat well and dish out in plates to serve.

Peppery Red Lentil Spread

Servings: 9

Cooking Time: 25 Minutes

Ingredients:

- 1 ½ cups red lentils, soaked overnight and drained
- 4 ½ cups water
- 1 sprig rosemary
- 2 bay leaves
- 2 roasted peppers, seeded and diced
- 1 shallot, chopped
- 2 cloves garlic, minced
- 1/4 cup olive oil
- 2 tablespoons tahini
- Sea salt and ground black pepper, to taste

Directions:

1.   Add the red lentils, water, rosemary and bay leaves to a saucepan and bring to a boil over high heat. Then, turn the heat to a simmer and continue to cook for 20 minutes or until tender.

2.   Place the lentils in a food processor.

3.   Add in the remaining ingredients and process until everything is well incorporated.

4.   Bon appétit!

Nutrition Info: Per Serving: Calories: 193; Fat: 8.5g; Carbs: 22.3g; Protein: 8.5g

Nice Spiced Cherry Cider

Servings: 16

Cooking Time: 4 Hours

Ingredients:

- 2 cinnamon sticks, each about 3 inches long
- 6-ounce of cherry gelatin
- 4 quarts of apple cider

Directions:

1. Using a 6-quarts slow cooker, pour the apple cider and add the cinnamon stick.

2. Stir, then cover the slow cooker with its lid. Plug in the cooker and let it cook for 3 hours at the high heat setting or until it is heated thoroughly.

3. Then add and stir the gelatin properly, then continue cooking for another hour.

4. When done, remove the cinnamon sticks and serve the drink hot or cold.

Nutrition Info: , Calories:100 Cal, Carbohydrates:0g, Protein:0g, Fats:0g, Fiber:0g.

Cookie Dough Milkshake

Servings: 2

Cooking Time: 0 Minute

Ingredients:

- 2 tablespoons cookie dough
- 5 dates, pitted
- 2 teaspoons chocolate chips
- 1/2 teaspoon vanilla extract, unsweetened
- 1/2 cup almond milk, unsweetened
- 1 ½ cup almond milk ice cubes

Directions:

1. Place all the ingredients in the order in a food processor or blender and then pulse for 2 to 3 minutes at high speed until smooth.

2. Pour the milkshake into two glasses and then serve with some cookie dough balls.

Nutrition Info: Calories: 208 Cal; Fat: 9 g: Carbs: 30 g; Protein: 2 g; Fiber: 2 g

Eggplant & Roasted Tomato Farro Salad

Servings: 3

Cooking Time: 1 Hour 30 Minutes

Ingredients:

- 4 small eggplants
- 1 ½ cups chopped cherry tomatoes
- ¾ cup uncooked faro
- 1 tablespoon olive oil
- 1 minced garlic clove
- ½ cup rinsed and drained chickpeas
- 1 tablespoon basil
- 1 tablespoon arugula
- ½ teaspoon salt and ground black pepper
- 1 tablespoon vinegar
- ½ cup toasted pine nuts

Directions:

1.   Preheat the oven at 300f temperature and prepare a baking sheet. Place cherry tomatoes on the baking liner and drizzle olive oil, salt, and black pepper on it and bake it for 30 to 35 minutes. Cook the faro in the salted water

for 30 to 40 minutes. Slice the eggplant and salt it and leave it for 30 minutes. After that, rinse it with water and dry it kitchen towel. Now peeled and sliced the eggplants. Now place these slices on the baking liner and season it with salt, pepper and olive oil. Bake it for to 20 minutes in the preheated oven at the 450f temperature. Flip the sides of eggplant and bake it for an additional 15 to 20 minutes. Bake the pine nuts for 5 minutes and sauté the garlic. Now mix all the ingredients in a bowl and serve it.

Nutrition Info: Carbohydrates 37g, protein 9g, fats 25g, calories 399.

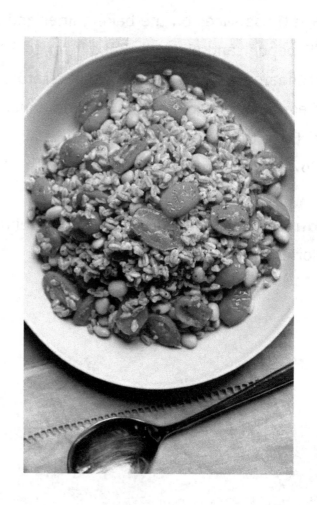

Simple Vegetable Broth

Servings: 4

Cooking Time: 45 Minutes

Ingredients:

- 3 tbsp olive oil
- 2 onions, quartered
- 2 carrots, chopped
- 1 cup celeriac, chopped
- 2 garlic cloves, unpeeled and crushed
- 6 cups water
- 2 tsp soy sauce
- ⅓ cup chopped fresh cilantro
- 1 bay leaf
- Salt to taste
- ½ tsp black peppercorns

Directions:

1. Warm the oil in a pot over medium heat. Place in onions, carrots, celeriac, and garlic. Cook for 5 minutes until softened. Pour in water, soy sauce, cilantro, bay

leaf, and peppercorns. Bring to a boil, lower the heat and simmer uncovered for 30 minutes.

2. Let cool for a few minutes, then pour over a strainer into a pot. Divide between glass mason jars and allow to cool completely. Seal and store in the fridge up to 5 days or 1 month in the freezer.

Grilled Tofu Mayo Sandwiches

Servings: 2

Cooking Time: 15 Minutes

Ingredients:

- ¼ cup tofu mayonnaise
- 2 slices whole-grain bread
- ¼ cucumber, sliced
- ½ cup lettuce, chopped
- ½ tomato, sliced
- 1 tsp olive oil, divided

Directions:

1.   Spread the vegan mayonnaise over a bread slice, top with the cucumber, lettuce and tomato and finish with the other slice. Heat the oil in a skillet over medium heat. Place the sandwich and grill for 3 minutes, then flip over and cook for a further 3 minutes. Cut the sandwich in half and serve.

Classic Onion Relish

Servings: 6

Cooking Time: 35 Minutes

Ingredients:

- 4 tablespoons vegan butter
- 1 pound red onions, peeled and sliced
- 4 tablespoons granulated sugar
- 4 tablespoons white vinegar
- 1 ½ cups boiling water
- 1 teaspoon sea salt
- 1 teaspoon mustard seeds
- 1 teaspoon celery seeds

Directions:

1.   In a frying pan, melt the butter over medium-high heat. Then, sauté the onions for about 8 minutes, stirring frequently to ensure even cooking.

2.   Add in the sugar and continue sautéing for 5 to 6 minutes more. Add in the vinegar, boiling water, salt, mustard seeds and celery seeds.

3.   Turn the heat to a simmer and continue to cook, covered, for about 20 minutes.

4.   Remove the lid and continue to simmer until all the liquid has evaporated. Bon appétit!

Nutrition Info: Per Serving: Calories: 118; Fat: 7.9g; Carbs: 11.3g; Protei

Jalapeno Rice Noodles

Servings: 4

Cooking Time: 25 Minutes

Ingredients:

- ¼ cup soy sauce
- 1 tablespoon brown sugar
- 2 teaspoons sriracha
- 3 tablespoons lime juice
- 8 oz rice noodles
- 3 teaspoons toasted sesame oil
- 1 package extra-firm tofu, pressed
- 1 onion, sliced
- 2 cups green cabbage, shredded
- 1 small jalapeno, minced
- 1 red bell pepper, sliced
- 1 yellow bell pepper, sliced
- 3 garlic cloves, minced
- 3 scallions, sliced
- 1 cup Thai basil leaves, roughly chopped
- Lime wedges for serving

Directions:

1.   Fill a suitably-sized pot with salted water and boil it on high heat.

2.   Add pasta to the boiling water and cook until it is al dente, then rinse under cold water.

3.   Put lime juice, soy sauce, sriracha, and brown sugar in a bowl then mix well.

4.   Place a large wok over medium heat then add 1 teaspoon sesame oil.

5.   Toss in tofu and stir for minutes until golden-brown.

6.   Transfer the golden-brown tofu to a plate and add 2 teaspoons oil to the wok.

7.   Stir in scallions, garlic, peppers, cabbage, and onion.

8.   Sauté for 2 minutes, then add cooked noodles and prepared sauce.

9.   Cook for 2 minutes, then garnish with lime wedges and basil leaves.

10.   Serve fresh.

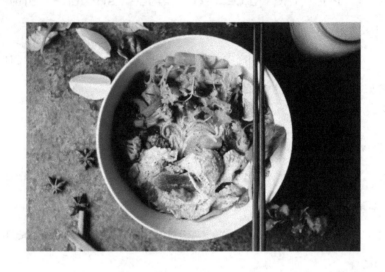

Spicy Broccoli in Pecan Pesto

Servings: 4

Cooking Time: 15 Minutes

Ingredients:

- 1 pound broccoli florets
- 2 cups chopped fresh basil
- ¼ cup olive oil
- 4 garlic cloves
- ½ cup pecans
- 1 tsp chili powder

Directions:

1. Place water in a pot and add the broccoli. Bring to a boil and steam for 5 minutes. In a blender, put basil, olive oil, garlic, pecans, and chili powder. Pulse until everything is blended. Drain the broccoli and mix in the basil sauce; toss to coat. Serve right away.

Pesto Mushroom Pizza

Servings: 4

Cooking Time: 40 Minutes

Ingredients:

- 2 tbsp flax seed powder
- ½ cup tofu mayonnaise
- ¾ cup whole-wheat flour
- 1 tsp baking powder
- 1 cup sliced mixed mushrooms
- 2 tbsp olive oil
- 1 tbsp basil pesto
- ½ cup red pizza sauce
- ¾ cup grated plant-based Parmesan

Directions:

1.   Preheat the oven to 350 F.

2.   In a medium bowl, mix the flax seed powder with 6 tbsp water and allow thickening for 5 minutes to make the flax egg. Mix in the tofu mayonnaise, whole-wheat flour, baking powder, and salt until dough forms. Spread

the dough on a pizza pan and bake in the oven for 10 minutes or until the dough sets.

3.　　In a medium bowl, mix the mushrooms, olive oil, basil pesto, salt, and black pepper. Remove the pizza crust spread the pizza sauce on top. Scatter mushroom mixture on the crust and top with plant-based Parmesan cheese. Bake further until the cheese melts and the mushrooms soften, 10 to 15 minutes. Remove the pizza, slice and serve.

Grilled Zucchini with Spinach Avocado Pesto

Servings: 4

Cooking Time: 20 Minutes

Ingredients:

- 3 oz spinach, chopped
- 1 ripe avocado, chopped
- Juice of 1 lemon
- 1 garlic clove, minced
- 2 oz pecans
- Salt and black pepper to taste
- ¾ cup olive oil
- 2 zucchini, sliced
- 1 tbsp fresh lemon juice
- 2 tbsp melted plant butter
- 1 ½ lb tempeh slices

Directions:

1.   Place the spinach in a food processor along with the avocado, lemon juice, garlic, and pecans. Blend until smooth and then, season with salt and black pepper. Add

the olive oil and process a little more. After, pour the pesto into a bowl and set aside.

2. Place zucchini in a bowl. Season with the remaining lemon juice, salt, black pepper, and the plant butter. Also, season the tempeh with salt and black pepper, and brush with olive oil. Preheat a grill pan and cook both the tempeh and zucchini slices until browned on both sides. Plate the tempeh and zucchini, spoon some pesto to the side, and serve immediately.

Pistachio Watermelon Steak

Servings: 4

Cooking Time: 10 Minutes

Ingredients:

- Microgreens
- Pistachios chopped
- Malden sea salt
- 1 tbsp. olive oil, extra virgin
- 1 watermelon
- Salt to taste

Directions:

1. Begin by cutting the ends of the watermelon.

2. Carefully peel the skin from the watermelon along the white outer edge.

3. Slice the watermelon into 4 slices, approximately 2 inches thick.

4. Trim the slices, so they are rectangular in shape approximately 2 xinches.

5. Heat a skillet to medium heat add 1 tablespoon of olive oil.

6.   Add watermelon steaks and cook until the edges begin to caramelize.

7.   Plate and top with pistachios and microgreens.

8.   Sprinkle with Malden salt.

9.   Serve warm and enjoy!

Nutrition Info: Calories: 67 Carbohydrates: 3.8 g Proteins: 1.6 g Fats: 5.9 g

Parsley Carrots & Parsnips

Servings: 4

Cooking Time: 25 Minutes

Ingredients:

- 2 tbsp plant butter
- ½ pound carrots, cut lengthways
- ½ pound parsnips, cut lengthways
- Salt and black pepper to taste
- ½ cup Port wine
- ¼ cup chopped fresh parsley

Directions:

1.   Melt the butter in a skillet over medium heat. Place in carrots and parsnips and cook for 5 minutes, stirring occasionally. Sprinkle with salt and pepper. Pour in Port wine and ¼ cup water. Lower the heat and simmer for minutes. Uncover and increase the heat. Cook until forms a syrupy sauce. Remove to a bowl and serve garnished with parsley.

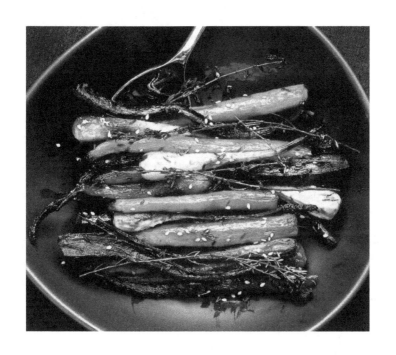

Raspberry Protein Shake

Servings: 1

Cooking Time: 5 Minutes

Ingredients:

- ¼ avocado
- 1 c. raspberries, frozen
- 1 scoop protein powder
- ½ c. almond milk
- Ice cubes

Directions:

1. In a high-speed blender add all the ingredients and blend until lumps of fruit disappear.

2. Add two to four ice cubes and blend to your desired consistency.

3. Serve immediately and enjoy!

Nutrition Info: Calories: 756 Carbohydrates: 80.1 g Proteins: 27.6 g Fats: 40.7 g

Rice Pudding with Currants

Servings: 4

Cooking Time: 45 Minutes

Ingredients:

- 1 ½ cups water
- 1 cup white rice
- 2 ½ cups oat milk, divided
- 1/2 cup white sugar
- A pinch of salt
- A pinch of grated nutmeg
- 1 teaspoon ground cinnamon
- 1/2 teaspoon vanilla extract
- 1/2 cup dried currants

Directions:

1.   In a saucepan, bring the water to a boil over medium-high heat. Immediately turn the heat to a simmer, add in the rice and let it cook for about 20 minutes.

2. Add in the milk, sugar and spices and continue to cook for minutes more, stirring constantly to prevent the rice from sticking to the pan.

3. Top with dried currants and serve at room temperature. Bon appétit!

Nutrition Info: Per Serving: Calories: 423; Fat: 5.3g; Carbs: 85g; Protein: 8.8g

Chocolate Rye Porridge

Servings: 4

Cooking Time: 10 Minutes

Ingredients:

- 2 cups rye flakes
- 2 ½ cups almond milk
- 2 ounces dried prunes, chopped
- 2 ounces dark chocolate chunks

Directions:

1. Add the rye flakes and almond milk to a deep saucepan; bring to a boil over medium-high. Turn the heat to a simmer and let it cook for 5 to 6 minutes.

2. Remove from the heat. Fold in the chopped prunes and chocolate chunks, gently stir to combine.

3. Ladle into serving bowls and serve warm.

4. Bon appétit!

Nutrition Info: Per Serving: Calories: 460; Fat: 13.1g; Carbs: 72.2g; Protein: 15g

Sweet Cornbread Muffins

Servings: 8

Cooking Time: 30 Minutes

Ingredients:

- 1 cup all-purpose flour
- 1 cup yellow cornmeal
- 1 teaspoon baking powder
- 1 teaspoon baking soda
- 1 teaspoon kosher salt
- 1/2 cup sugar
- 1/2 teaspoon ground cinnamon
- 1 1/2 cups almond milk
- 1/2 cup vegan butter, melted
- 2 tablespoons applesauce

Directions:

1. Start by preheating your oven to 420 degrees F. Now, spritz a muffin tin with a nonstick cooking spray.

2. In a mixing bowl, thoroughly combine the flour, cornmeal, baking soda, baking powder, salt, sugar and cinnamon.

3. Gradually add in the milk, butter and applesauce, whisking constantly to avoid lumps.

4. Scrape the batter into the prepared muffin tin. Bake your muffins for about 25 minutes or until a tester inserted in the middle comes out dry and clean.

5. Transfer them to a wire rack to rest for minutes before unmolding and serving. Bon appétit!

Nutrition Info: Per Serving: Calories: 311; Fat: 13.7g; Carbs: 42.3g; Protein: 4.5g

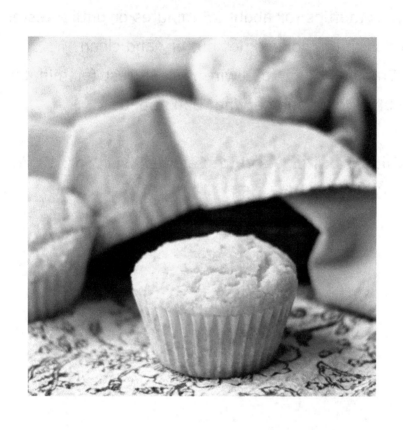

Tangy Chickpea Soup with a Hint of Lemon

Servings: 6

Cooking Time: 30 Minutes

Ingredients:

- 2 cups of freshly diced onion
- 3 freshly minced large garlic cloves
- Water
- ½ cup of freshly diced celery
- ¾ teaspoon of sea salt
- Freshly ground black pepper to taste
- 1 teaspoon of mustard seeds
- ½ teaspoon of dried oregano
- 1 teaspoon of cumin seeds
- ½ teaspoon of paprika
- 1 ½ teaspoons of dried thyme
- 3 ½ cups of cooked chickpeas
- 1 cup of dried red lentils
- 3 cups of vegetable stock
- 2 dried bay leaves
- 2 cups of freshly chopped tomatoes or zucchini
- 2 cups of water

- ¼ to 1/3 cup of fresh lemon juice

Directions:

1. Put a large pot on the stove on medium heat.
2. Add onion, water, salt, celery, garlic, pepper, cumin, and mustard seeds along with thyme, oregano, and paprika. Stir everything to combine well.
3. Cover the pot and cook for about 7 minutes, stirring occasionally.
4. Rinse the lentils.
5. Add the lentils along with 2 ½ cups of chickpeas, zucchini/tomatoes, stock, bay leaves, and water. Stir everything to combine well.
6. Increase the heat to bring to a boil.
7. Once the ingredients start to boil, cover the pot, lower the heat, and simmer for 20-25 minutes.
8. You will know that the soup is ready when the lentils are tender.
9. After removing the bay leaves, add the lemon juice.

10.   Once the ingredients have cooled down, use a hand blender to puree the ingredients, but keep a somewhat coarse texture instead of having a smooth puree.

11.   Add the remaining chickpeas. Taste the soup and adjust the salt, pepper, and lemon juice to taste.

12.   Enjoy this amazing soup with your favorite bread.

Classic Pecan Pie

Servings: 4

Cooking Time: 50 Minutes

Ingredients:

- For the piecrust:
- 4 tbsp flax seed powder + 12 tbsp water
- 1/3 cup whole-wheat flour + more for dusting
- ½ tsp salt
- ¼ cup plant butter, cold and crumbled
- 3 tbsp pure malt syrup
- 1 ½ tsp vanilla extract
- For the filling:
- 3 tbsp flax seed powder + 9 tbsp water
- 2 cups toasted pecans, coarsely chopped
- 1 cup light corn syrup
- ½ cup pure date sugar
- 1 tbsp pure pomegranate molasses
- 4 tbsp plant butter, melted
- ½ tsp salt
- 2 tsp vanilla extract

Directions:

1.   Preheat the oven to 350 F and grease a large pie pan with cooking spray.

2.   In a medium bowl, mix the flax seed powder with water and allow thickening for 5 minutes. Do this for the filling's flax egg too in a separate bowl.

3.   In a large bowl, combine the flour and salt. Add the plant butter and using an electric hand mixer, whisk until crumbly. Pour in the crust's flax egg, maple syrup, vanilla, and mix until smooth dough forms.

4.   Flatten the dough on a flat surface, cover with plastic wrap, and refrigerate for 1 hour.

5.   After, lightly dust a working surface with flour, remove the dough onto the surface, and using a rolling pin, flatten the dough into a 1-inch diameter circle.

6.   Lay the dough on the pie pan and press to fit the shape of the pan. Use a knife to trim the edges of the pan. Lay a parchment paper on the dough, pour on some baking beans and bake in the oven until golden brown, 15 to 20 minutes. Remove the pan from the oven, pour out the baking beans, and allow cooling.

7.   In a large bowl, mix the filling's flax egg, pecans, corn syrup, date sugar, pomegranate molasses, plant butter, salt, and vanilla. Pour and spread the mixture on the piecrust. Bake further for 20 minutes or until the filling sets. Remove from the oven, decorate with more pecans, slice, and cool. Slice and serve.

Nutrition Info: al infoper serving: Calories 99; Fats 59.8g; Carbs 117.6 g; Protein 8g

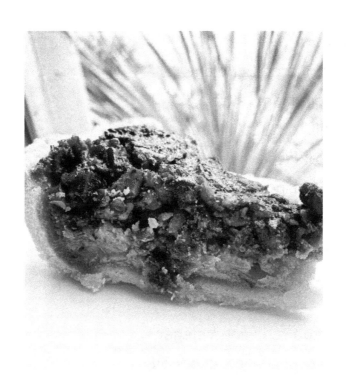

Grilled Eggplant with Pecan Butter Sauce

Servings: 2

Cooking Time: 31 Minutes

Ingredients:

- Marinated Eggplant:
- 1 eggplant, sliced
- Salt to taste
- 4 tablespoons olive oil
- ¼ teaspoon smoked paprika
- ¼ teaspoon ground turmeric
- Black Bean and Pecan Sauce:
- ⅓ cup vegetable broth
- ⅓ cup red wine
- ⅓ cup red wine vinegar
- 1 large shallot, chopped
- 1 teaspoon ground coriander
- 2 teaspoons minced cilantro
- ½ cup pecan pieces, toasted
- 2 roasted garlic cloves
- 4 small banana peppers, seeded, and diced
- 8 tablespoons butter

- 1 tablespoon chives, chopped
- 1 (15.5 ounce) can black beans, rinsed and drained
- Salt and black pepper to taste
- 1 teaspoon fresh lime juice

Directions:

1. In a saucepan, add broth, wine, vinegar, shallots, coriander, cilantro and garlic.

2. Cook while stirring for minutes on a simmer.

3. Meanwhile blend butter with chives, pepper, and pecans in a blender.

4. Add this mixture to the broth along with salt, lime juice, black pepper, and beans.

5. Mix well and cook for minutes.

6. Rub the eggplant with salt and spices.

7. Prepare and set up the grill over medium heat.

8. Grill the eggplant slices for 6 minutes per side.

9. Serve the eggplant with prepared sauce.

10. Enjoy.

Cremini Mushroom Risotto

Servings: 3

Cooking Time: 20 Minutes

Ingredients:

- 3 tablespoons vegan butter
- 1 teaspoon garlic, minced
- 1 teaspoon thyme
- 1 pound Cremini mushrooms, sliced
- 1 ½ cups white rice
- 2 ½ cups vegetable broth
- 1/4 cup dry sherry wine
- Kosher salt and ground black pepper, to taste
- 3 tablespoons fresh scallions, thinly sliced

Directions:

1. In a saucepan, melt the vegan butter over a moderately high flame. Cook the garlic and thyme for about minute or until aromatic.

2. Add in the mushrooms and continue to sauté until they release the liquid or about 3 minutes.

3. Add in the rice, vegetable broth and sherry wine. Bring to a boil; immediately turn the heat to a gentle simmer.

4. Cook for about 15 minutes or until all the liquid has absorbed. Fluff the rice with a fork, season with salt and pepper and garnish with fresh scallions.

5. Bon appétit!

Nutrition Info: Per Serving: Calories: 513; Fat: 12.5g; Carbs: 88g; Protein: 11.7g

Sweet Potato & Black Bean Protein Salad

Servings: 2

Cooking Time: 0 Minutes

Ingredients:

- 1 cup dry black beans
- 4 cups of spinach
- 1 medium sweet potato
- 1 cup purple onion, chopped
- 2 tbsp. olive oil
- 2 tbsp. lime juice
- 1 tbsp. minced garlic
- ½ tbsp. chili powder
- ¼ tsp. cayenne
- ¼ cup parsley
- Salt and pepper to taste

Directions:

1. Prepare the black beans according to the method.
2. Preheat the oven to 400°F.

3.   Cut the sweet potato into ¼-inch cubes and put these in a medium-sized bowl. Add the onions, 1 tablespoon of olive oil, and salt to taste.

4.   Toss the ingredients until the sweet potatoes and onions are completely coated.

5.   Transfer the ingredients to a baking sheet lined with parchment paper and spread them out in a single layer.

6.   Put the baking sheet in the oven and roast until the sweet potatoes are starting to turn brown and crispy, around 40 minutes.

7.   Meanwhile, combine the remaining olive oil, lime juice, garlic, chili powder, and cayenne thoroughly in a large bowl, until no lumps remain.

8.   Remove the sweet potatoes and onions from the oven and transfer them to the large bowl.

9.   Add the cooked black beans, parsley, and a pinch of salt.

10.   Toss everything until well combined.

11.   Then mix in the spinach, and serve in desired portions with additional salt and pepper.

12.   Store or enjoy!

Basic Homemade Tahini

Servings: 16

Cooking Time: 10 Minutes

Ingredients:
- 10 ounces sesame seeds, hulled
- 3 tablespoons canola oil
- 1/4 teaspoon kosher salt

Directions:

1.   Toast the sesame seeds in a nonstick skillet for about 4 minutes, stirring continuously. Cool the sesame seeds completely.

2.   Transfer the sesame seeds to the bowl of your food processor. Process for about 1 minute.

3.   Add in the oil and salt and process for a further 4 minutes, scraping down the bottom and sides of the bowl.

4.   Store your tahini in the refrigerator for up to 1 month. Bon appétit!

Nutrition Info: Per Serving: Calories: 135; Fat: 13.4g; Carbs: 2.2g; Protein: 3.6g

Pecan And Apricot Butter

Servings: 16

Cooking Time: 15 Minutes

Ingredients:

- 2 ½ cups pecans
- 1/2 cup dried apricots, chopped
- 1/2 cup sunflower oil
- 1 teaspoon bourbon vanilla
- 1/4 teaspoon ground anise
- 1/2 teaspoon cinnamon
- 1/8 teaspoon grated nutmeg
- 1/8 teaspoon salt

Directions:

1.   In your food processor or a high-speed blender, pulse the pecans until ground. Then, process the pecans for 5 minutes more, scraping down the sides and bottom of the bowl.

2.   Add in the remaining ingredients.

3.   Run your machine for a further 5 minutes or until the mixture is completely creamy and smooth. Enjoy!

Nutrition Info: Per Serving: Calories: 163; Fat: 17g; Carbs: 2.5g; Protein: 1.4g

Spicy Cilantro and Mint Chutney

Servings: 9

Cooking Time: 10 Minutes

Ingredients:

- 1 ½ bunches fresh cilantro
- 6 tablespoons scallions, sliced
- 3 tablespoons fresh mint leaves
- 2 jalapeno peppers, seeded
- 1/2 teaspoon kosher salt
- 2 tablespoons fresh lime juice
- 1/3 cup water

Directions:

1. Place all the ingredients in the bowl of your blender or food processor.

2. Then, combine the ingredients until your desired consistency has been reached.

3. Bon appétit!

Nutrition Info: Per Serving: Calories: 15; Fat: 0g; Carbs: 0.9g; Protein: 0.1g

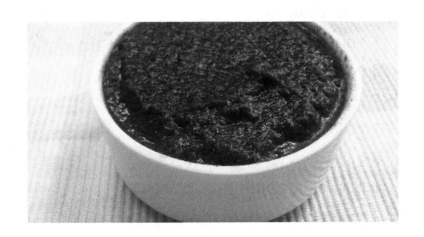

Pomegranate Bell Peppers & Eggplants

Servings: 4

Cooking Time: 40 Minutes

Ingredients:

- ½ cup olive oil
- 1 onion, chopped
- 3 eggplants, cut into chunks
- 1 red pepper, chopped
- 1 yellow bell pepper, chopped
- 2 garlic cloves, minced
- 1 hot chili, seeded and minced
- 2 tbsp pomegranate molasses
- ½ cup orange juice
- 2 tsp pure date sugar
- 1 ripe peach, chopped
- ½ cup finely chopped fresh cilantro

Directions:

1.   Heat the oil in a skillet over medium heat. Place the onion and sauté for 5 minutes. Add in eggplants, bell peppers, garlic, and chili. Cook for minutes. Stir in

pomegranate molasses, orange juice, sugar, salt, and pepper. Bring to a boil, then lower the heat and simmer for 20 minutes, until the liquid reduce. Top with peach and cilantro and serve right away.

Mushroom Steak

Servings: 8

Cooking Time: 1 Hour

Ingredients:

- 1 tbsp. of the following:
- fresh lemon juice
- olive oil, extra virgin
- 2 tbsp. coconut oil
- 3 thyme sprigs
- 8 medium Portobello mushrooms
- For Sauce:
- 1 ½ t. of the following:
- minced garlic
- minced peeled fresh ginger
- 2 tbsp. of the following:
- light brown sugar
- mirin
- ½ c. low-sodium soy sauce

Directions:

1.   For the sauce, combine all the sauce ingredients, along with ¼ cup water into a little pan and simmer to cook. Cook using a medium heat until it reduces to a glaze, approximately to 20 minutes, then remove from the heat.

2.   For the mushrooms, bring the oven to 350 heat setting.

3.   Using a skillet, melt coconut oil and olive oil, cooking the mushrooms on each side for about minutes.

4.   Next, arrange the mushrooms in a single layer on a sheet for baking and season with lemon juice, salt, and pepper.

5.   Carefully slide into the oven and roast for minutes. Let it rest for 2 minutes.

6.   Plate and drizzle the sauce over the mushrooms.

7.   Enjoy.

Nutrition Info: Calories: 87 Carbohydrates: 6.2 g Proteins: 3 g Fats: 6.2 g

Grilled Carrots with Chickpea Salad

Servings: 8

Cooking Time: 10 Minutes

Ingredients:

- Carrots
- 8 large carrots
- 1 tablespoon oil
- 1 ½ teaspoon salt
- 1 teaspoon dried oregano
- 1 teaspoon dried thyme
- 2 teaspoon paprika powder
- 1 ½ tablespoon soy sauce
- ½ cup of water
- Chickpea Salad
- 14 oz canned chickpeas
- 3 medium pickles
- 1 small onion
- A big handful of lettuce
- 1 teaspoon apple cider vinegar
- ½ teaspoon dried oregano
- ½ teaspoon salt

- Ground black pepper, to taste
- ½ cup vegan cream

Directions:

1. Toss the carrots with all of its ingredients in a bowl.

2. Thread one carrot on a stick and place it on a plate.

3. Preheat the grill over high heat.

4. Grill the carrots for 2 minutes per side on the grill.

5. Toss the ingredients for the salad in a large salad bowl.

6. Slice grilled carrots and add them on top of the salad.

7. Serve fresh.

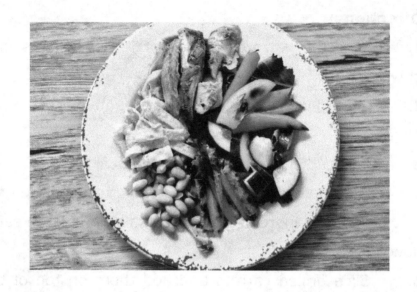

Parsley Pumpkin Noodles

Servings: 4

Cooking Time: 15 Minutes

Ingredients:

- ¼ cup plant butter
- ½ cup chopped onion
- 1 pound pumpkin, spiralized
- 1 bunch kale, sliced
- ¼ cup chopped fresh parsley
- Salt and black pepper to taste

Directions:

1.   Mel the butter in a skillet over medium heat. Place the onion and cook for 3 minutes. Add in pumpkin and cook for another 7-8 minutes. Stir in kale and cook for another 2 minutes, until the kale wilts. Sprinkle with parsley, salt and pepper and serve.

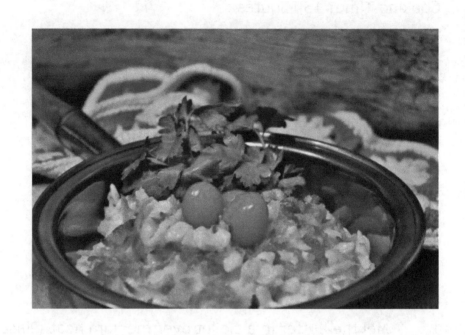

Sweet Potato Croutons Salad

Servings: 4

Cooking Time: 20 Minutes

Ingredients:

- 12s-ounce baked sweet potato, skin-on, cut into pieces
- 2 mandarin oranges, peeled, segmented, halved
- 1-pound mixed salad greens and vegetables
- 1 sweet apple, cored, diced, air fried
- 2 tablespoons balsamic vinegar
- 1/3 cup pomegranate seeds

Directions:

1. Switch on the air fryer, insert the fryer basket, then shut it with the lid, set the frying temperature 350 degrees F, and let it preheat for 5 minutes.

2. Meanwhile, prepare sweet potatoes, and for this, dice them into small pieces.

3. Open the preheated fryer, place sweet potatoes in it in a single layer, spray with olive oil, close the lid and

cook for 20 minutes until golden brown and cooked, shaking halfway.

4.   When done, the air fryer will beep, open the lid, and then transfer sweet potato croutons to a salad bowl.

5.   Add remaining ingredients, gently stir until combined, and then serve.

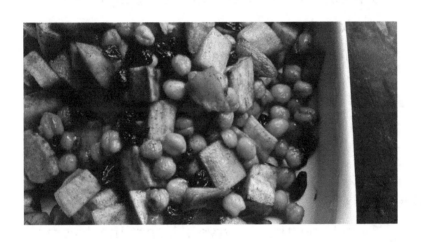

Rainbow Vegetables Salad

Servings: 4

Cooking Time: 20 Minutes

Ingredients:

- 1 medium red bell pepper, deseeded, diced
- 1/2 of medium sweet onion, cut into wedges
- 1 medium yellow summer squash, diced
- 1 zucchini, diced
- 4 ounces mushrooms, halved
- 1/3 teaspoon ground black pepper
- 2/3 teaspoon salt
- 1 tablespoon olive oil

Directions:

1.   Switch on the air fryer, insert the fryer basket, then shut it with the lid, set the frying temperature 350 degrees F, and let it preheat for 5 minutes.

2.   Meanwhile, take a large bowl, place all the vegetables in it, drizzle with oil, season with salt and black pepper and toss until coated.

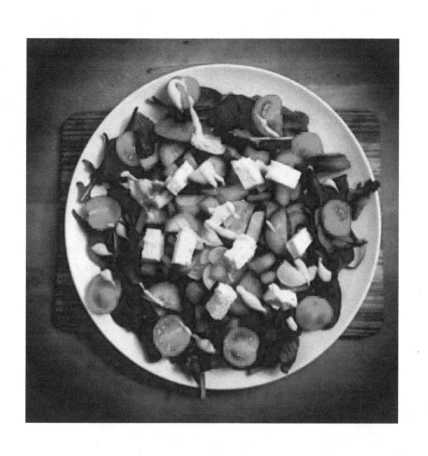